SELF CARE FOR NEW *Mums*

THE LITTLE THINGS THAT MATTER MOST

SELINA PERI

Contents

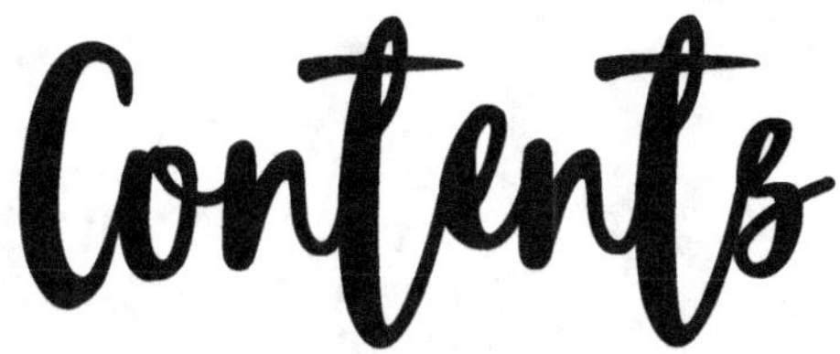

Introduction

What is Self-Care

Why is Self-Care important to mums

How this book helps

MORNING RITUAL

BUILDING YOUR MUM TRIBE

PILATES IN PAJAMAS

REIGNITING YOUR PASSIONS

FINDING ZEN

FROM YES TO NO

CONFESSIONS OF A CAFFEINATED MUM

SETTING HEALTHY BOUNDARIES

DIGITAL DETOX

SWEATPANTS TO SUPERWOMAN

COMMUNICATE OPENLY

NAPTIME POWER

MASTERING YOUR ZZZZ

SWEET SURRENDER

MUM GUILT

FROM MESSY TO MARVELLOUS

LAUGHTER YOGA FOR MUMS

EMBRACING YOUR IMPERFECTIONS

RECHARGE YOUR SPIRIT

SNEAKY SNACKS

HAVE A JOURNAL

CALL YOUR BEST FRIEND

A DISTRACTION FREE COFFEE

Introduction

Becoming a mother was a profound transformation that altered the course of my life in ways I could never have anticipated. The moment I held my newborn in my arms, I was overwhelmed with love, joy, and an huge sense of responsibility. The experience of bringing a new life into the world was awe-inspiring, but it also brought challenges that stretched me to my limits.

In those early days of motherhood, as I adjusted to sleepless nights, endless diaper changes, and the constant demands of a tiny, fragile being, I found myself immersed in a world of nurturing and caregiving.

It was a world I had eagerly embraced, but in the process, I had unwittingly neglected one vital aspect of well-being: myself.

The idea of self-care felt like an extravagant luxury I couldn't afford, a frivolous indulgence in the face of the all-encompassing role of being a mother. The days turned into weeks, and the weeks into months, during which I put my own needs on the back burner, convinced that my child's well-being was the only priority.

As time went on, the signs of self-neglect became increasingly evident. I was exhausted, physically and emotionally drained, and my once-vibrant spirit felt dimmed. I found myself snapping at my loved ones, wrestling with a rollercoaster of emotions, and struggling to regain a sense of equilibrium. I was, in essence, running on empty.

Then, one day, amidst the chaos and exhaustion, something changed. It wasn't a moment of grand revelation, but a subtle awakening, a whisper from within that said, "You deserve care too." That whisper marked the beginning of my journey to self-care—a journey that would transform my life, my relationship with my child, and the way I approached motherhood.

Through my experiences, I hope to inspire and guide you on your own path to self-care, reminding you that nurturing yourself is not a selfish act but a necessary one. It is my firm belief that by caring for ourselves, we become better mothers, partners, and individuals. So, come with me on this journey, and let's discover the incredible transformation that can happen when we make self-care a priority in the beautiful chaos of motherhood.

Selina x

What is Self-Care?

A holistic and deliberate approach, self-care for mothers focuses on fostering well-being by identifying and meeting physical, emotional, and mental needs. In the face of the responsibilities of motherhood, it entails making thoughtful decisions and setting aside time for pursuits that help with rest, renewal, and a sense of personal fulfilment.

Mums can engage in a variety of self-care activities, ranging from straightforward daily routines to intricate rituals, all aimed at supporting a balanced and healthy lifestyle.

This can involve doing things like practising mindfulness, making things, taking up hobbies, taking pauses, getting enough sleep, keeping up with friends, and doing things that make you happy and fulfilled.

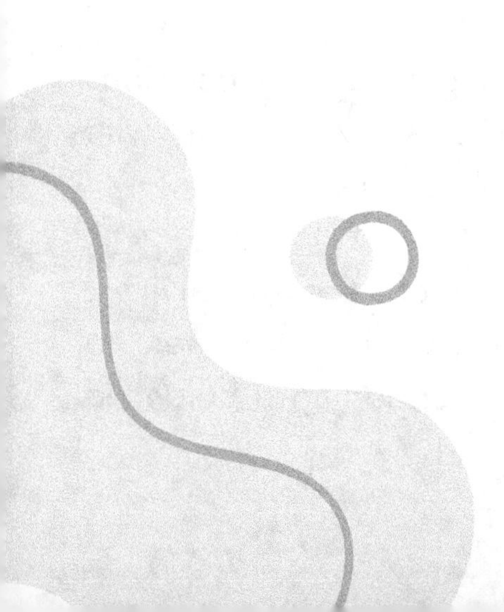

Why is Self-Care important to mums?

For mothers, self-love is essential for a number of reasons:

Resilience: Being a mother comes with many obstacles and unknowns. Resilience is built on self-love, which enables mothers to overcome obstacles, disappointments, and the unavoidable stressors that come with being a parent.

Emotional well-being: is improved when self-love is prioritised. Mothers who love themselves are better able to handle stress, worry, and the emotional burden of taking care of others.

Mums are the main role models that their children look up to. Children learn the value of self-respect, healthy boundaries, and self-care when they see adults modelling self-love.

Physical Well-Being: Taking good care of oneself is a sign of love for oneself. It guarantees that mothers have the vitality and energy required to fulfil the responsibilities of parenthood.

Managing Roles: Mothers frequently juggle being a partner, caregiver, and career. Self-love promotes a sense of fulfilment, avoids burnout, and helps to maintain a balance between these responsibilities.

Enhanced Empathy and Patience: Mothers who value self-care are better able to control their emotions. This improves empathy and patience, which in turn fosters a more loving and supportive atmosphere for them and their family.

How this book helps

This book is like a warm hug for your spirit; it's a gentle guide to help you through the wonderful and challenging journey of motherhood, with an emphasis on taking care of the most vital person involved: yourself.

It serves as a reminder that being a mum entails treating yourself with kindness rather than offering advice on how to be a mother.

It inspires you to value the times that make you feel good, accept the messiness, and take delight in the little things in life. It's a friend that will encourage you to take some time for yourself, whether it's a hot cup of tea, a read-aloud passage, or some alone time for contemplation.

MORNING
Ritual

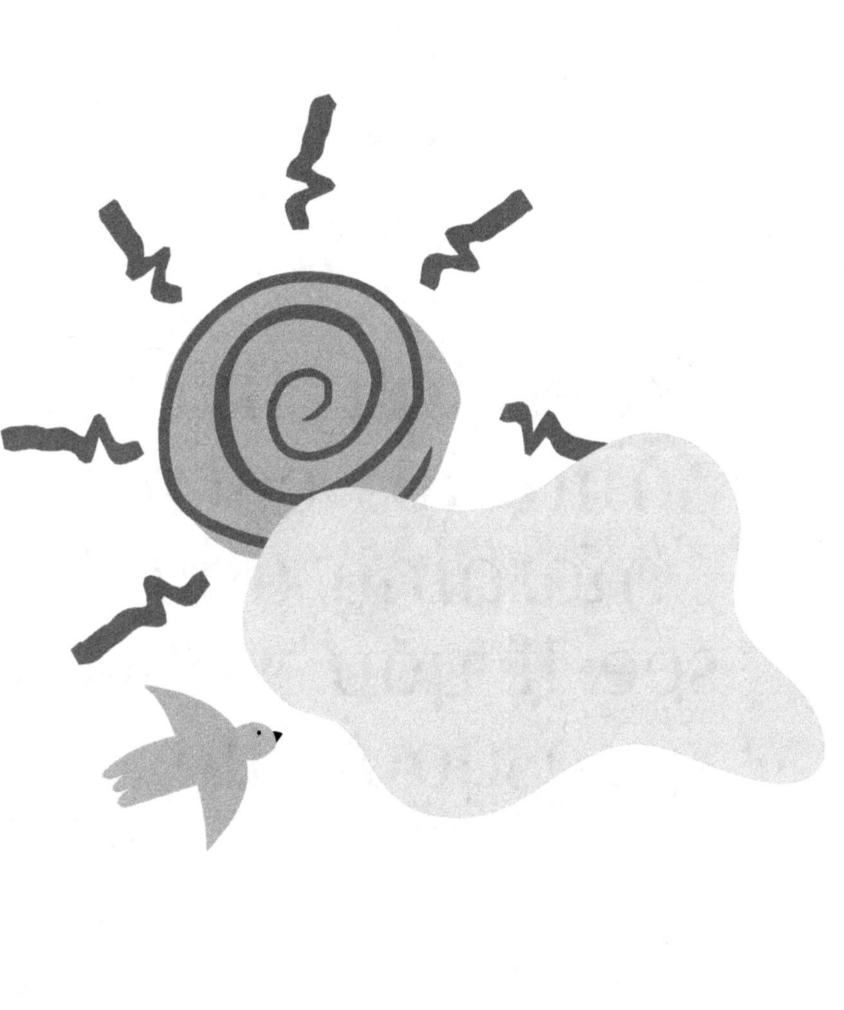

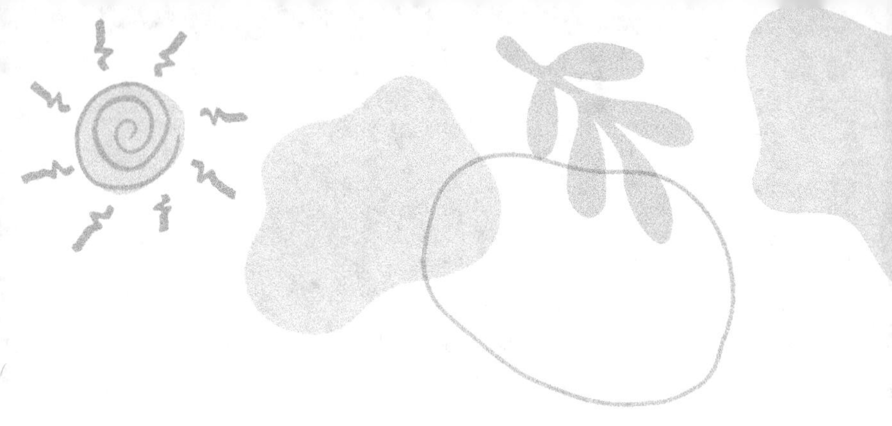

meditate five
minutes each
morning and
see if you wake
up your life

One way to start your day off right is to take a moment each morning to express your thanks. Think about the things in your life for which you are grateful for a few minutes. By engaging in this easy exercise, you can change your perspective from concentrating on what is lacking or negative to seeing the richness and happiness all around you.

As you carry this grateful attitude with you throughout your daily activities, it sets the tone for a day full of optimism and increased well-being.

It's the act of putting your physical and mental health first while still accepting convenience and comfort.

Envision waking up, having a glass of water to refresh your body and starting a little Pilates exercise that energises you for the day.

BUILDING YOUR
Mum Tribe

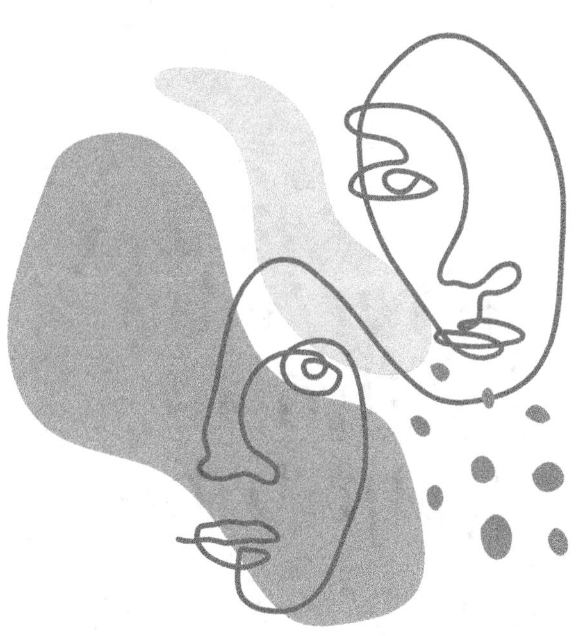

your vibe
attracts
your tribe

Creating your mum tribe is similar to building your own support network—a network of other mothers who are familiar with the highs and lows of the motherhood experience.

Your mum tribe is there to participate in the happiness of your children's accomplishments, laugh with you over cereal spills, and offer support during trying times. They're your go-to people for helping you discover self-care moments because they understand how important it is to take a break and look after your own wellbeing.

You will plan play dates that involve adult talks, share self-care tips, and support one another during difficult times. It's not just a group; they are also your confidantes, friends, and supporters who help you on your self-care path.

PILATES IN
Pajamas

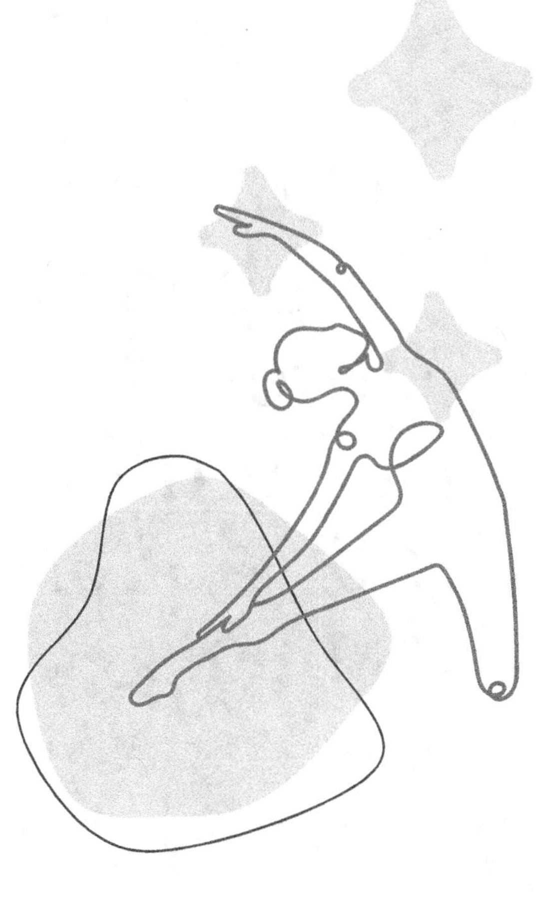

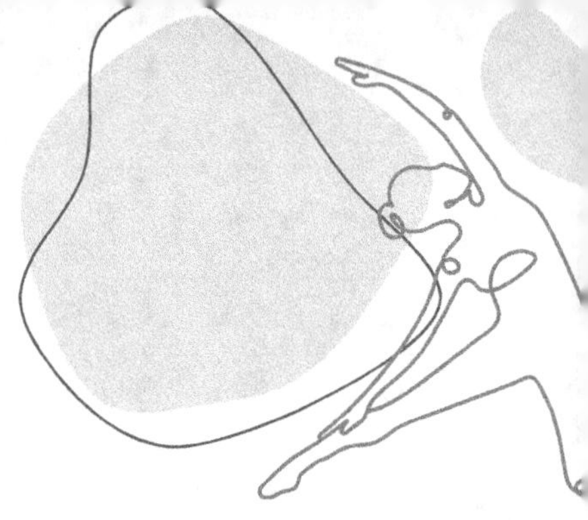

change
happens
through
movement
and motion
heals

It's the practice of embracing comfort and convenience while still prioritising your physical well-being. Imagine rolling out of bed, slipping into your comfiest pyjamas, and engaging in a gentle pilates routine that energises your body and mind.

No need for fancy workout gear or gym memberships – just you, your mat, and a commitment to self-care in the cosiest attire. It's a reminder that self-care can be as comfortable and inviting as your favourite pair of PJs, allowing you to tone your body and rejuvenate your spirit without the fuss. So, why not start your day with a dose of self-love?

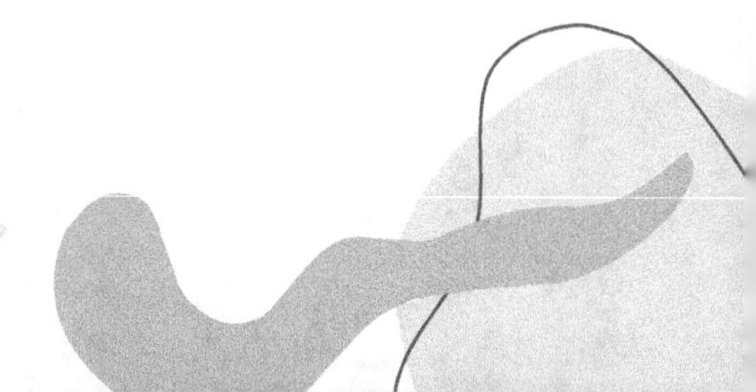

REIGNITING YOUR
Passions

04

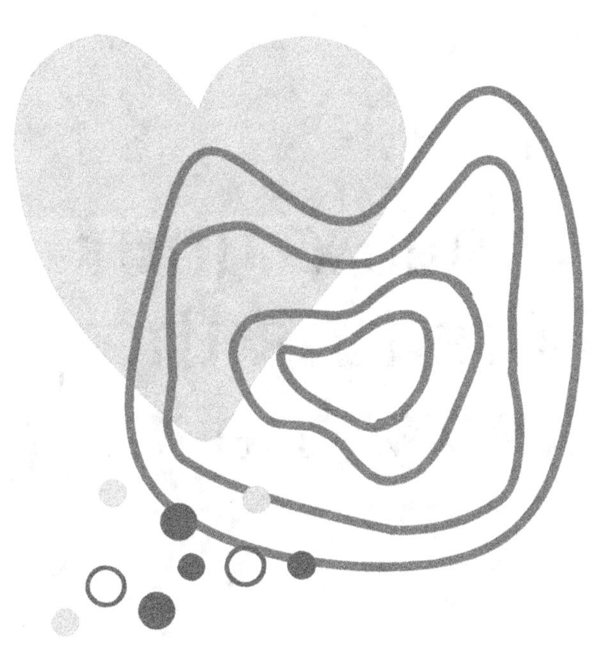

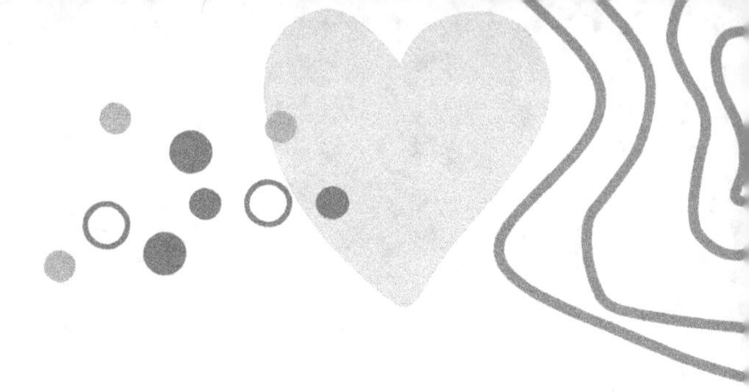

follow your
dreams they
know the way

This is your call to reignite the passion that defines who you are! Although motherhood is a wonderful experience, it's simple to get lost in the daily frenzy of diaper changes and baby giggling.

Finding your own passions and interests again, whether they are writing, dancing, painting, or something else entirely, is the focus of this chapter. It's about finding that inner spark again and recalling the aspirations and abilities that made your heart skip a beat before you entered the world of motherhood.

Self-care is fanning the flames of your soul as much as your physical needs. To rekindle your passions with an energy that can only come from a fulfilled and regenerated you, dust off that old instrument, pick up that novel you've forgotten, and get going.

FINDING

Zen

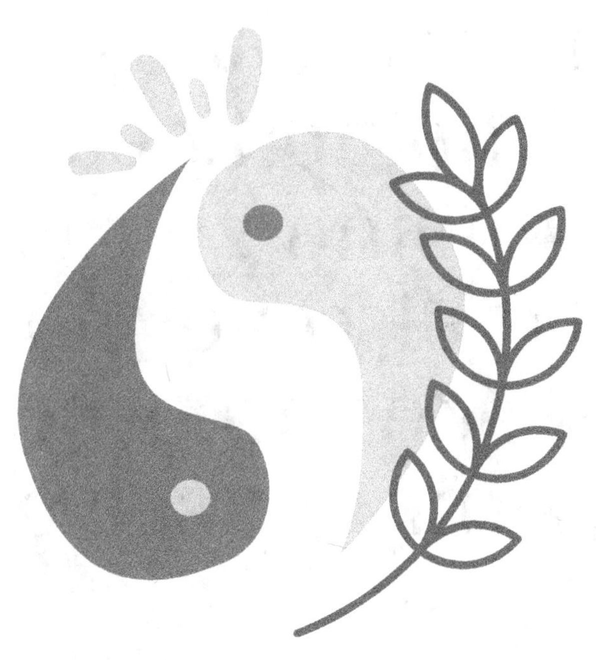

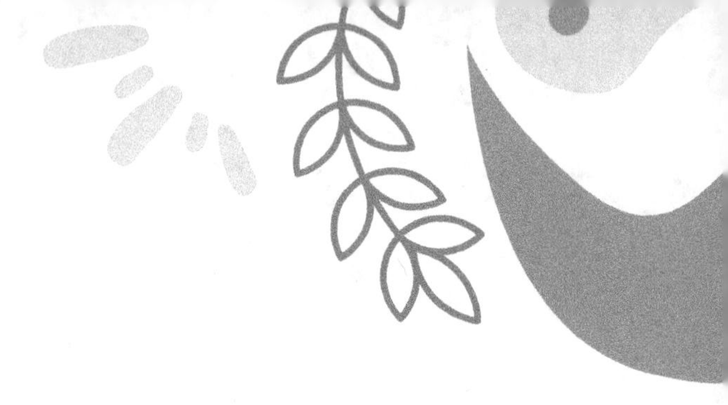

in the chaos of
motherhood;
finding zen is
like discovering a
hidden treasure
within ourselves.

It's about creating your sanctuary out of those ephemeral moments of silence. As a mother, I am aware of how life's clamour can occasionally smother our inner tranquillity. But somewhere amid the constant washing, tantrums, and changing of diapers is a calm place that's just waiting to be found. It's in the peaceful sighs, soft lullabies, and the sweet times when your child's hand catches your finger.

Let Go of Perfection: Remind yourself that not everything has to be picture-perfect; instead, find beauty in the flaws.

Nap Power: Take advantage of your baby's naptime to relax or engage in a pastime as your own little piece of personal zen.

Learn to Say No: Avoid overcommitting yourself by telling others no when you need more time to yourself.

Enjoy the Silence: When the house is quiet, try not to add more noise and instead, enjoy the tranquillity.

06

FROM

Yes To No

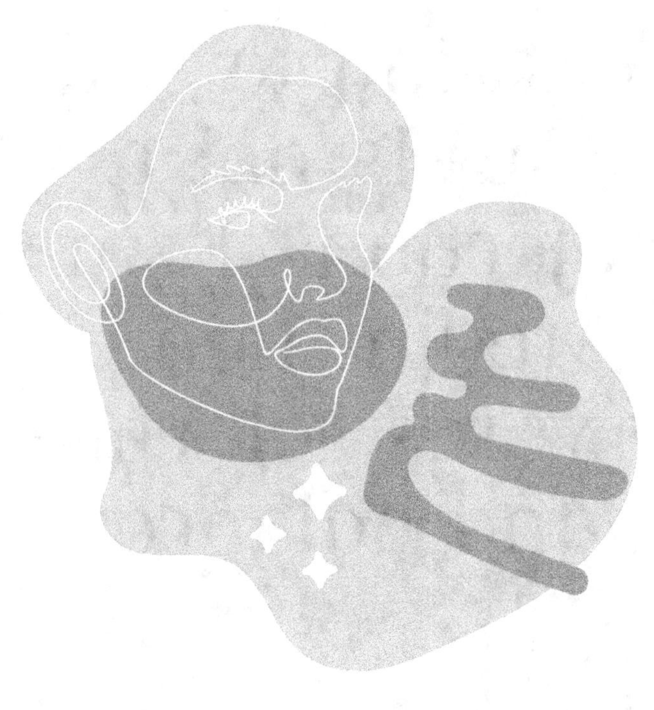

learning to say 'no' is not a rejection; it's a redirection towards self-care and balance

Being a mother makes saying "yes" seem natural. Our desire is to be there for our spouses, kids, and anybody else who needs us.

Saying "no" is a significant act of self-care, though. It's about maintaining your wellbeing and setting boundaries, not about being egotistical.

I've been there before, trying to be superwoman and fulfilling every request, but it just made me feel exhausted and overburdened.

It's critical to speak up for what you need and to put your priorities first. It can be freeing to say "no" when it's essential. This can free up time and energy for self-care, making you a happier and healthier mother.

CONFESSIONS OF A
Caffeinated Mum

in a world of diaper changes and sleepless nights; a cup of coffee is the secret elixir that keeps my mum-sanity intact

As a coffee-loving mom, I've learned that a simple coffee break can be a moment of respite, a chance to collect our thoughts, and an opportunity to savor a warm cup of comfort.

Oh the joy and challenges of parenting with a latte in hand, self-care isn't just about grand gestures but also the little moments of delight that help us find balance and nourish our well-being as we embrace the beautiful chaos of motherhood.

So, grab your coffee, chat to a friend, and confess the delightful ways we keep our mum-spirits high.

SETTING HEALTHY
Boundaries

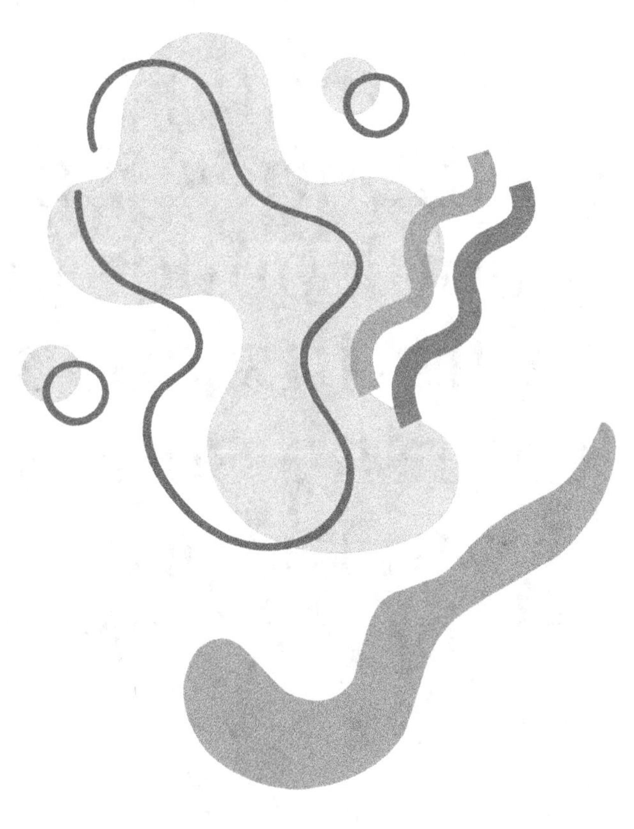

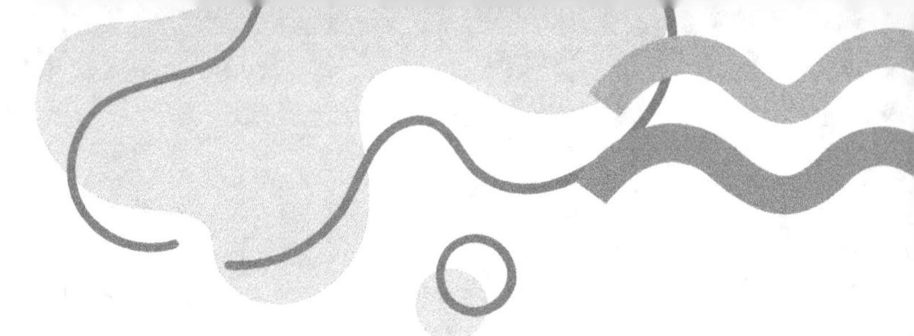

setting
boundaries isn't
about building
walls; it's about
creating spaces
where your
well-being thrives

As a mother, establishing healthy boundaries is an essential part of your self-care journey. It's similar to encircling your wellbeing with protection and making sure you have time to take care of yourself in spite of the responsibilities of parenting.

The following activities will assist you in creating and upholding these boundaries.

Establish Priorities: List the things that are most important to you as a mother and as a person. Your decision to set boundaries will be guided by your priorities.

Practice saying "no" to obligations or assignments that conflict with your priorities by practicing expressing "no" with grace. It's ok to politely decline when called for.

Share and Delegate Responsibilities: You don't have to handle everything by yourself. Assign parenting responsibilities and domestic chores to your spouse or ask.

Plan your "Me Time:" Make sure you schedule regular time for self-care and mark it as non-negotiable.

Digital
Detox

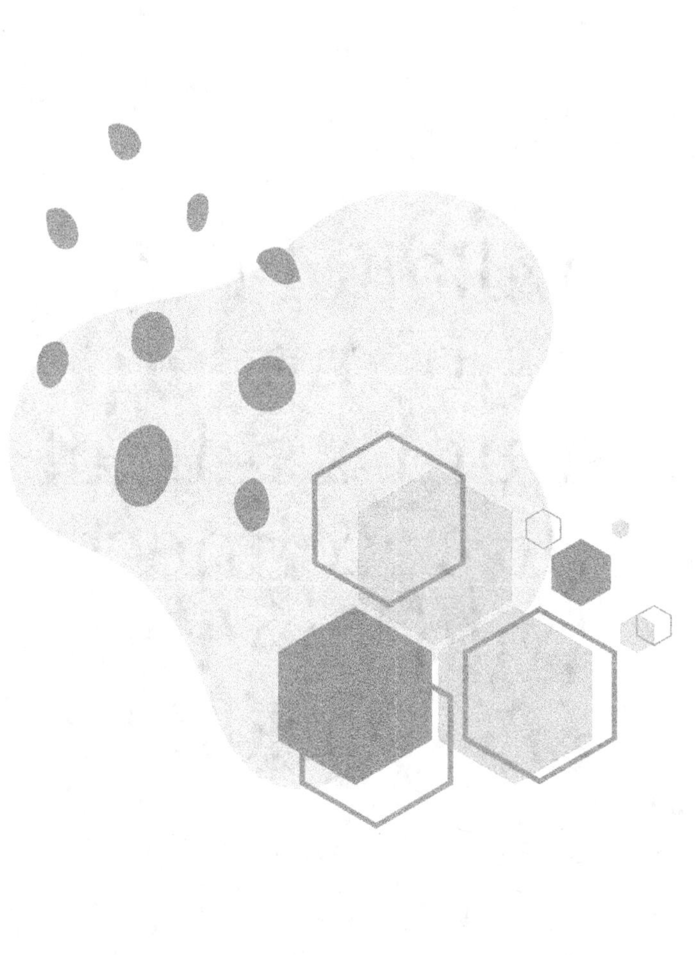

a digital detox
is a modern
mum's retreat
to reconnect
with the real
world

We get caught in the social media maze, notifications, and never-ending connectedness. However, the focus is on how crucial it is to disconnect, even for a brief period, in order to find time for self-care. Setting boundaries and taking back your presence in the present moment are more important than fully giving up on technology.

Imagine the delight of enjoying a quiet cup of tea, reading a book, or spending quality time with your kids without the interruption of devices. These times of detachment function as a kind of reset button, enabling you to refuel and become a more patient and present mother.

Sweatpants to *Superwoman*

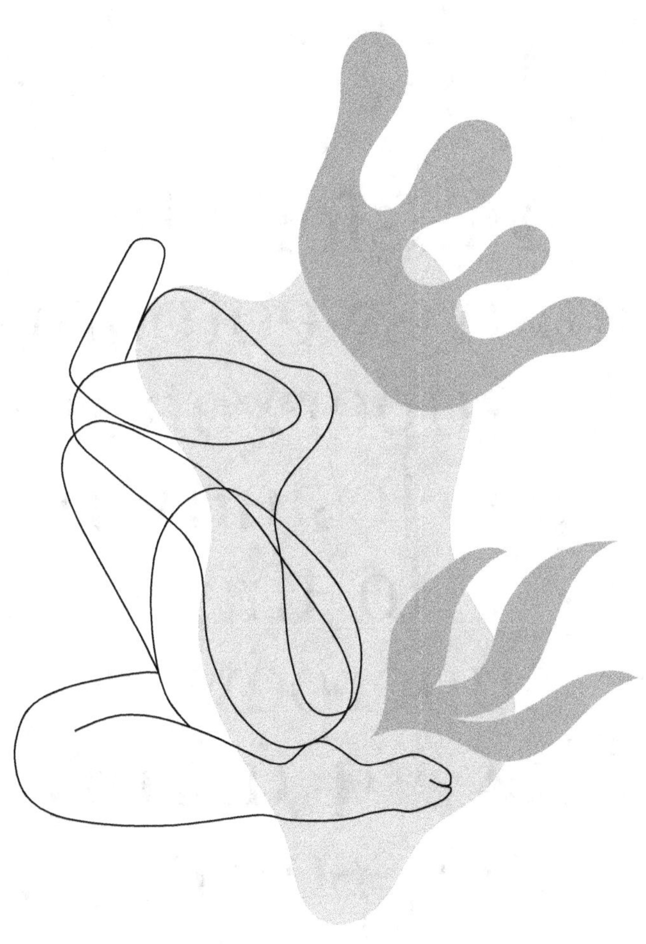

transforming
from sweatpants
to superwoman
is a testament
to the
superpowers
every mum
possesses

It's totally normal to embrace the comfort of sweatpants on days when you're a mum and wear them. But it's also important to keep in mind that beneath those soft exteriors is a superwoman who runs the family, raises her kids, and frequently balances employment and a plethora of other obligations.

Embrace your two selves: the carefree, comfortable you and the unstoppable, heroic mother. It's about setting aside some time to celebrate your successes, support your sense of self-worth, and keep in mind that you are superhuman in terms of tenacity, love, and willpower.

You're amazing, regardless of whether you're wearing sweatpants or a cape. Taking care of yourself and recognizing your strength is what self-care is all about. From your family's perspective, you are the true superhero.

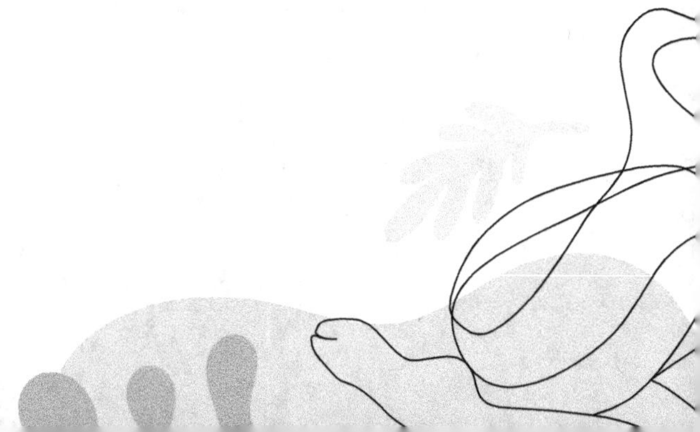

Communicate *Openly*

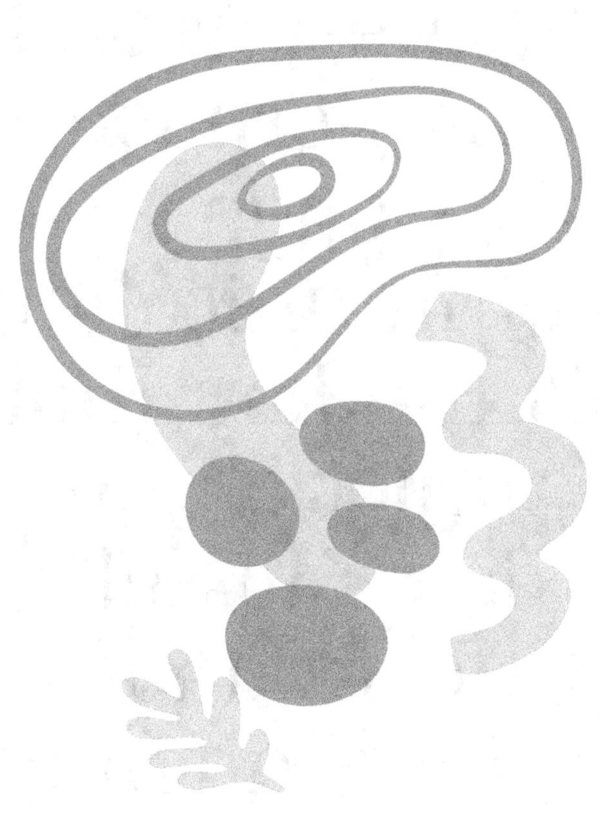

in the world of motherhood; open communication is the key that unlocks the doors to self-care and understanding.

In the path of motherhood, communication is essential, especially for recently arrived mothers. It's critical to communicate your needs, worries, and joys to yourself as well as to those you love. The following tips will assist you in prioritizing self-care and having honest conversations.

Discuss Your Feelings: Have a talk about your feelings as a new mother with your significant other or a reliable friend. It can be helpful to simply talk about your experiences sometimes.

Ask for Assistance: Never hesitate to seek for assistance when you need it. Communication is essential, whether it's for help with tasks or a respite from infant duty.

Establish Boundaries: Tell your loved ones when you take time for yourself. Your needs will be honoured thanks to this open discussion.

Celebrate Your Success: Talk about all your accomplishments, whether small and large, as a mother. Acknowledging your successes is a crucial component of self-care.

NAPTIME Power

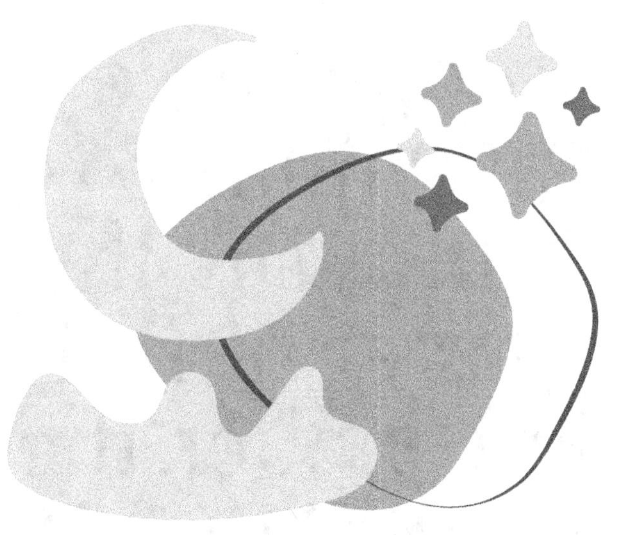

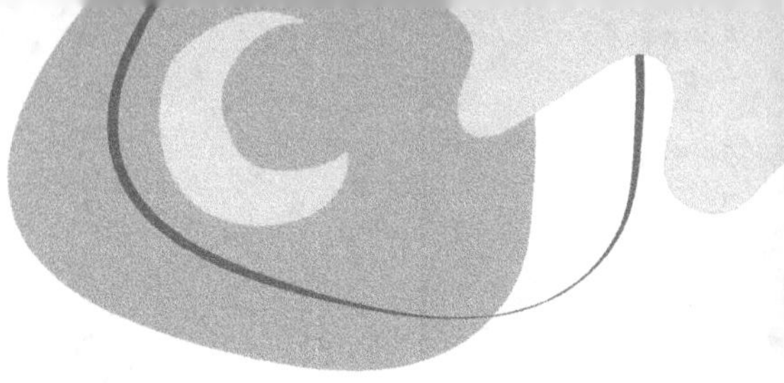

during naptime; a mum harnesses the power of rest to conquer the world of motherhood

This is your chance to rejuvenate, revitalize, and rediscover your vitality to tackle the rigors of parenthood.

As a mother, I've discovered that making the most of these peaceful times may have a profound impact. It's a time to take care of oneself, whether it's getting more rest, reading a nice book, doing yoga, or just relaxing with a cup of tea by yourself.

Your superhero cape and go-to tool for staying sane and strong amid the chaos of parenting is naptime power. Thus, take advantage of these times, accept the others, and utilize them to your advantage. It's necessary to be the best mother you can be it's not selfish.

MASTERING YOUR

ZZZZ

a well-rested mum is a superhero in disguise; ready to conquer the world of motherhood

In actuality, when you put rest first, you're not just ensuring that you receive a decent night's sleep; you're also providing yourself with the patience and energy necessary to meet the demands of motherhood with grace and enthusiasm.

As a mother, you are aware that getting enough sleep is like having a hidden weapon that will help you deal with any parenting difficulty and improve your attitude and creativity.

Taking care of yourself doesn't have to be complicated—just press the snooze button and become the supermum you were always intended to be.

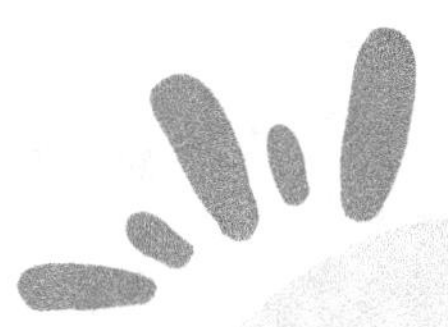

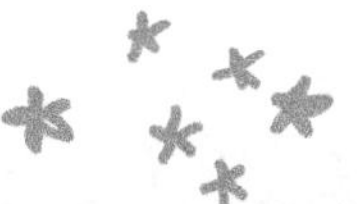

SWEET

Surrender

14

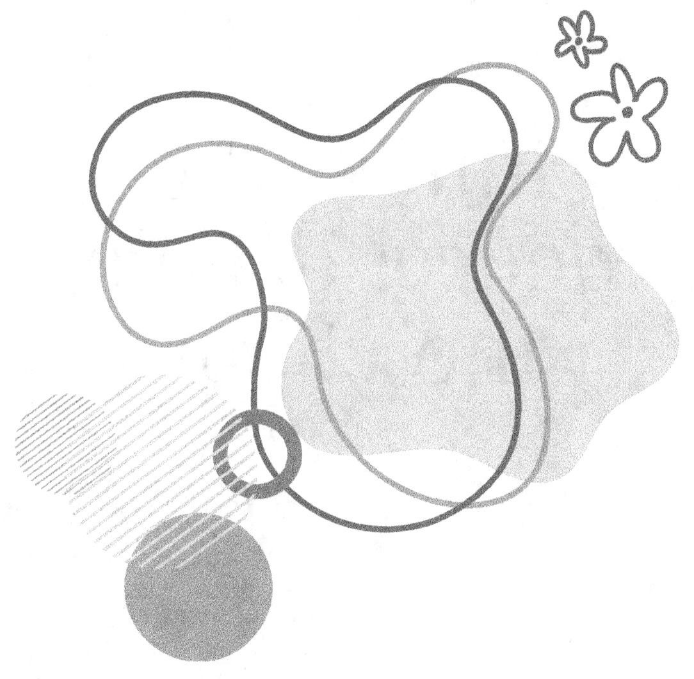

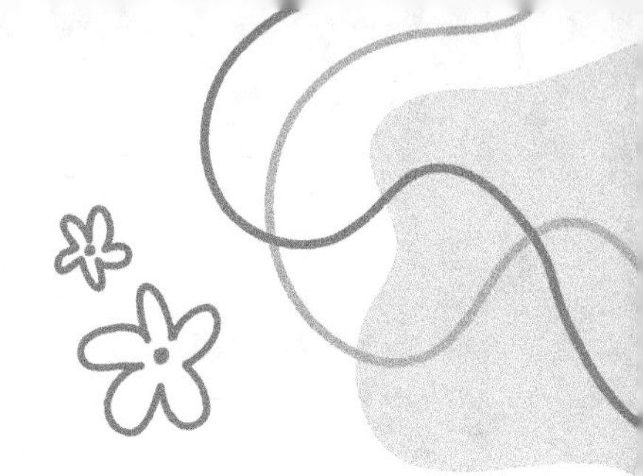

inhale the
peace; exhale
the chaos

Aromatherapy is a sensory-soothing form of self-care that is akin to a fragrant getaway into peace. Being a mother puts you in the delightful but taxing turmoil of raising children.

It provides an opportunity to indulge in the aromas that can elevate your spirits and soothe your mind.

Here's a gentle reminder that taking a moment to breathe in the relaxing air of lavender or relish the stimulating scent of citrus can be sufficient self-care. In the lovely chaos of parenthood, aromatherapy is your sensory haven where you may find moments of calm and renewal.

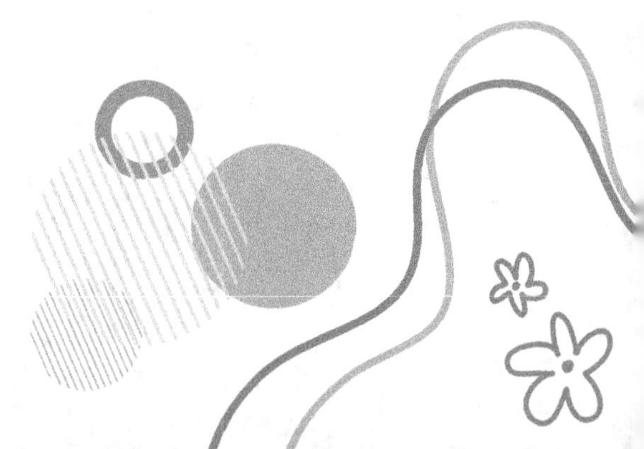

15

MUM

Guilt

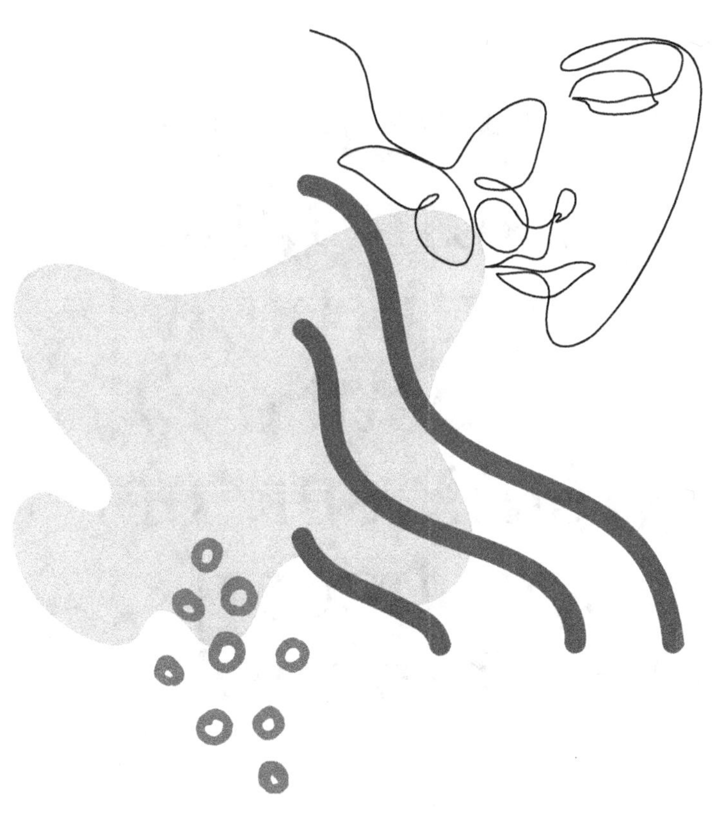

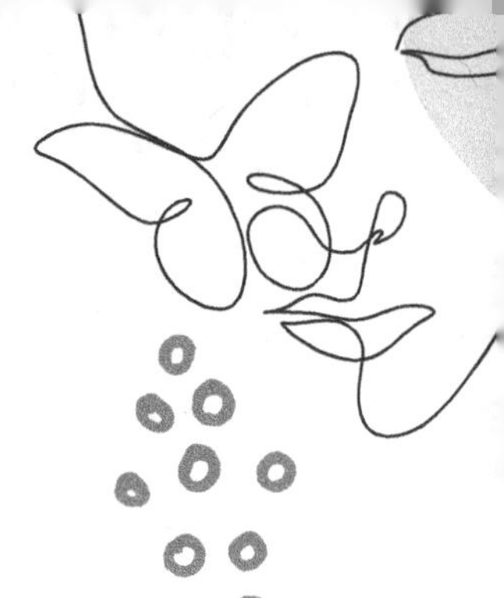

redefining mum guilt: let it be a gentle reminder; not a heavy burden

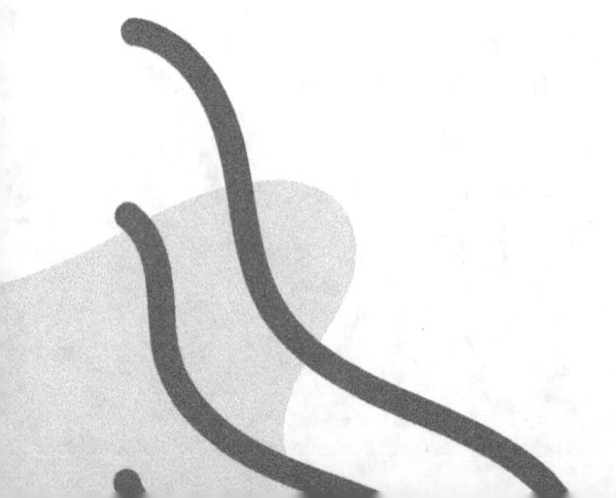

Practice: The Journal of Guilt

Spend a few minutes every day writing down any moments when you experienced motherhood guilt. Jot down the particular circumstance, your emotions, and your accompanying thoughts.

Examine your entries after a week of recording these moments. Any recurrent themes or trends?

Write down a more realistic and self-compassionate viewpoint for each occurrence. Respond to the guilt with compassion and reason.

How do you feel?

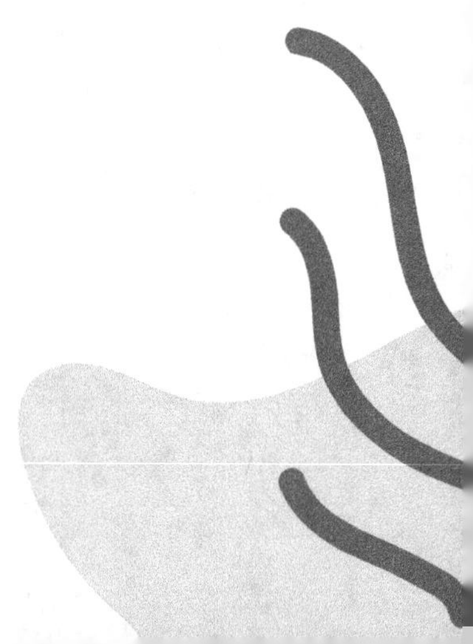

FROM MESSY
To Marvellous

life may be messy; but in the chaos; we find the most marvellous moments

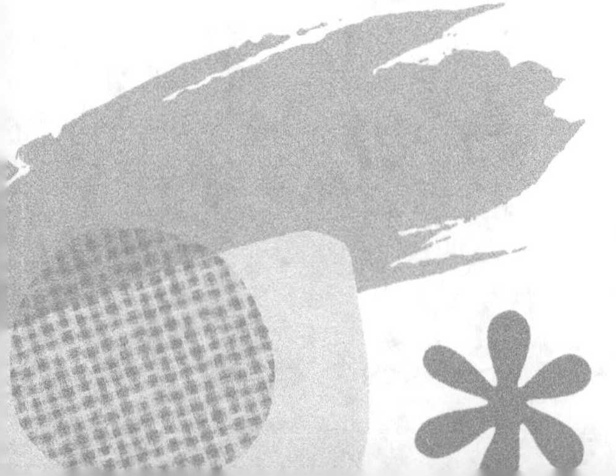

The beautiful chaos of parenthood, complete with anything from cereal spills to wall murals created by crayon drawings, is something that mothers frequently experience.

The trick is to change our viewpoint so that we may see the chaos as a blank canvas for amazing memories and as a reminder that self-care can still be successful even in the middle of chaos.

It's a reminder to accept the untidy times and understand that self-care is about nourishing your spirit in the midst of the lovely chaos that is parenting, not about attaining perfection.

So let's embrace the mess, take pleasure in the flaws, and learn that self-care is necessary even in the messiest of circumstances.

LAUGHTER YOGA
For Mums

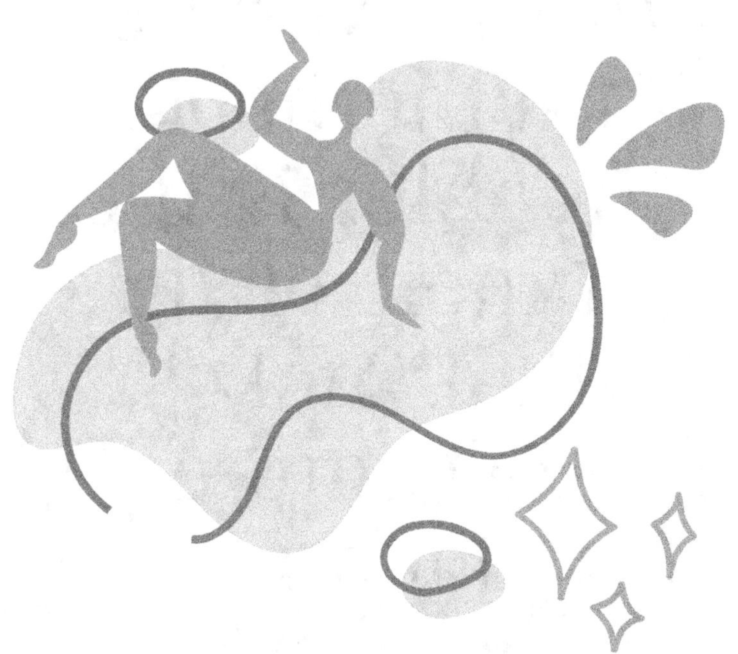

in the world of
motherhood;
laughter is the
magic elixir
that makes
self-care a
joyous
journey

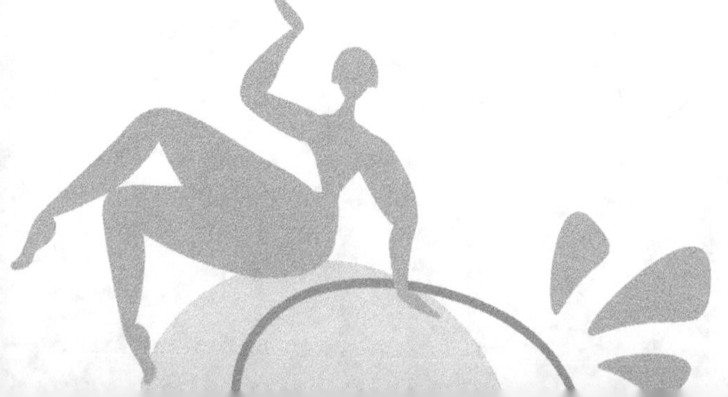

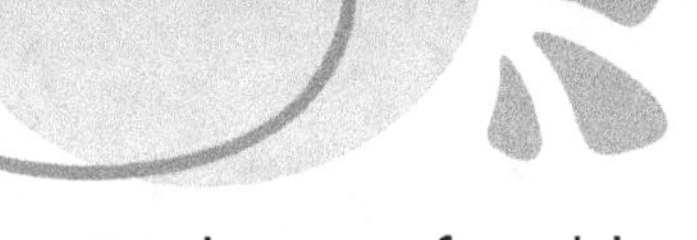

- Find a comfortable space, and with a mirror or without, stand, sit, or lie down.

- Start by taking a few deep breaths to relax.

- Now, begin to laugh! It might feel a little forced at first, but soon, the genuine giggles will emerge. You can even incorporate playful movements like clapping your hands or nodding your head to enhance the experience.

- Focus on the positive, humorous side of motherhood. Think about funny moments or the quirky things your kids do.

- After a few minutes, take a deep breath, and exhale slowly, allowing yourself to return to a calm state.

This is a fun and effective way to infuse your day with positivity and joy. It's a reminder that self-care doesn't always have to be serious; it can be filled with laughter and lightness, making your motherhood journey even more delightful!

18

EMBRACING YOUR
Imperfections

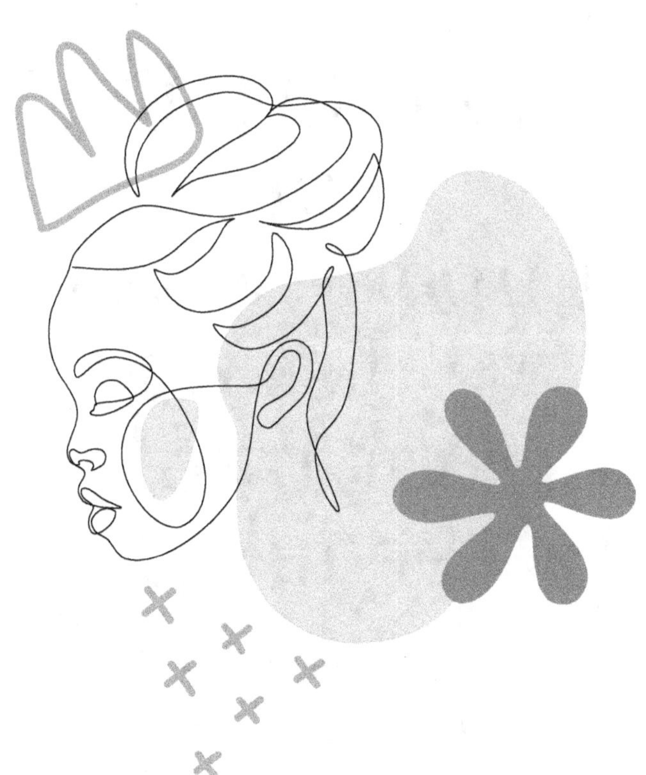

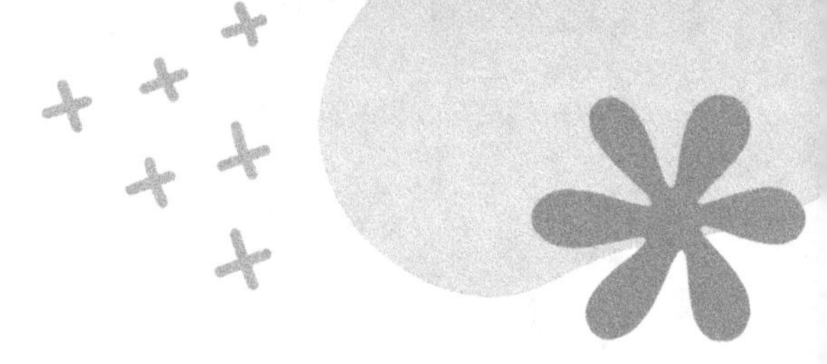

in embracing
our
imperfections;
we discover
our true
beauty

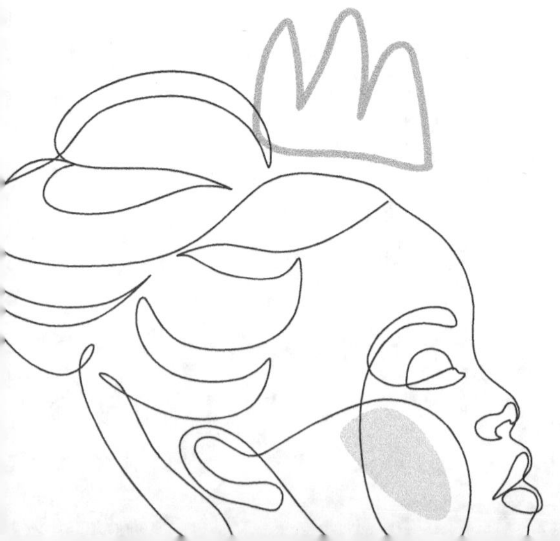

Although we mothers frequently aim for perfection, our true selves can be found in our flaws.

This chapter is an invitation to let go of the expectation of perfect parenting, realising that self-care is about taking care of our inner selves as much as our children.

It serves as a gentle reminder to accept our eccentricities, to make mistakes, and to experience moments of self-doubt.

We find freedom and the time to really take care of ourselves when we do this.

Therefore, let's embrace our flaws since they are signs of a lovely and authentic motherhood journey. When we accept ourselves as we are, flaws and all, self-care can begin.

RECHARGE YOUR *Spirit*

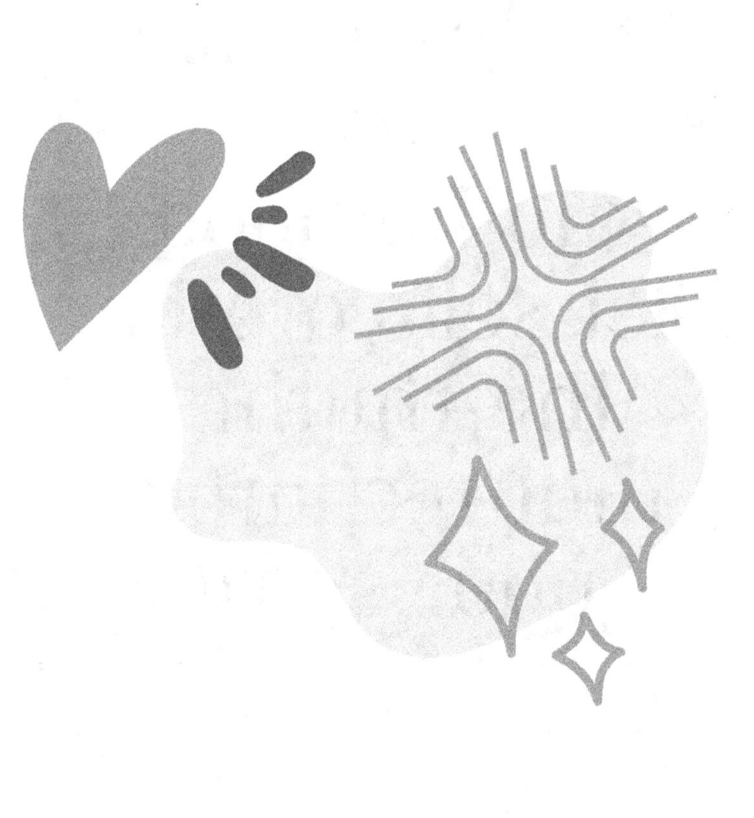

in the dance
of
motherhood;
let self-care be
the rhythm
that recharges
your spirit.

Motherhood is a beautiful journey, but it can also be demanding.

As mums, it's crucial to prioritise self-care to ensure we have the energy and resilience needed to navigate the challenges that come our way. Recharging your spirit is not just a luxury; it's a necessity. Let's explore some practical and rejuvenating ways to infuse your life with positivity and energy.

Gratitude Journal:
Dedicate a few minutes each day to jot down three things you're grateful for.

Reflect on the positive aspects of your life, even on challenging days. This practice helps shift your focus toward the uplifting elements, fostering a sense of gratitude.

Affirmation Practice:
Create a list of positive affirmations tailored to your needs.

Repeat these affirmations daily, especially in the morning or before bedtime. Affirmations can uplift your spirit and instil a positive mindset.

SNEAKY *Snacks*

20

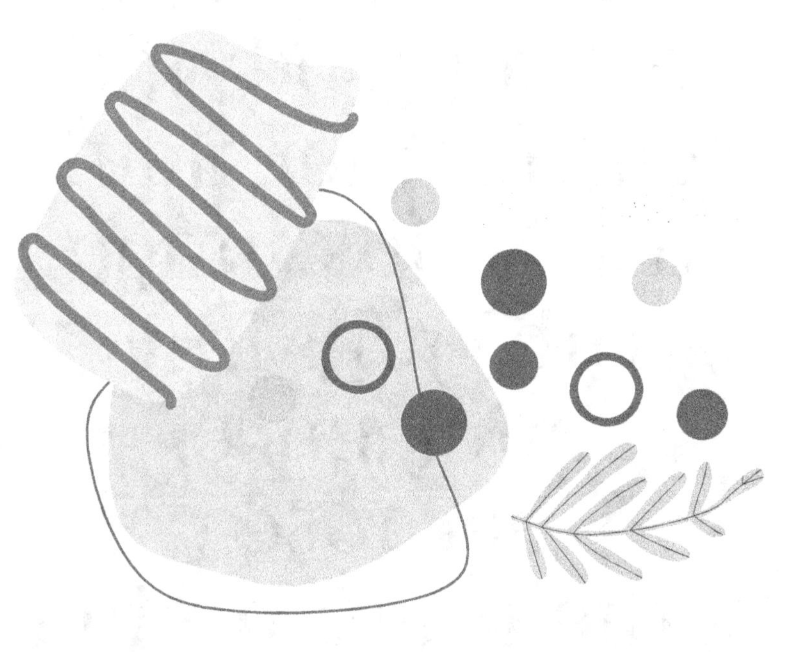

in the delightful dance between motherhood and self-care; let your taste buds tango with guilt-free indulgence. because sometimes; a little sweetness is the secret ingredient to a happy mum

In the process of practising self-care, we frequently forget that treating oneself doesn't always have to be expensive; sometimes, all it takes is the act of indulging in a guilt-free snack to feel better.

These dishes are quick, simple, and full of flavour that will take you to a blissful place, even if only for a little while. They are created with you in mind.

RECIPES
Blissful Banana Bites

Ingredients:
2 Ripe bananas
100g Dark chocolate (70% cocoa or higher)
Chopped nuts (almonds, walnuts, or pistachios)

Instructions:
Slice bananas into bite-sized pieces.
Melt dark chocolate in a microwave-safe bowl.
Dip banana slices in melted chocolate, then coat with chopped nuts.
Place on a tray lined with parchment paper and freeze for a heavenly treat.

Cocoa-Coconut Energy Bites

Ingredients:

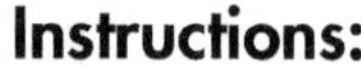

1 Cup rolled oats
2 tbsp unsweetened shredded coconut
1 tbsp cocoa powder
1 tbsp almond butter
Honey

Instructions:
Mix rolled oats, shredded coconut, and cocoa powder in a bowl.

Add honey and almond butter, combining until the mixture forms a dough.

Roll into bite-sized balls and refrigerate for a satisfying energy boost.

Remember, these treats are not just snacks—they're mini celebrations of self-love. So, indulge, savour, and embrace the joy of guilt-free mum treats!

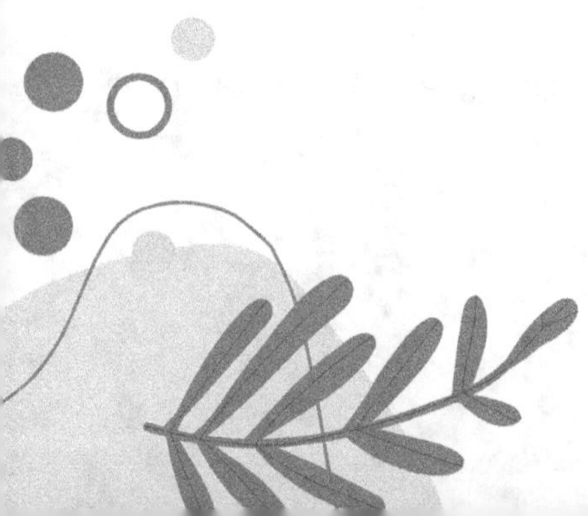

HAVE A

Journal

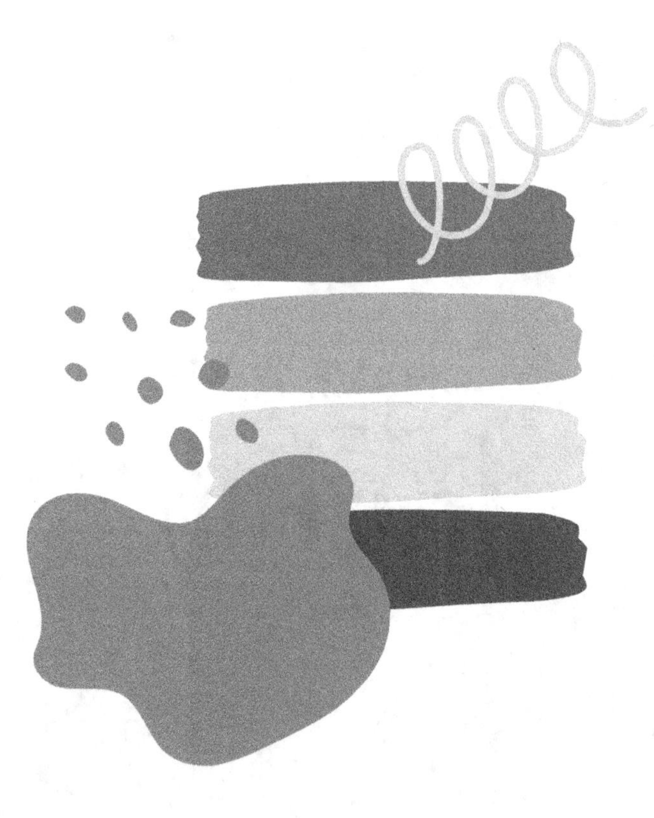

in the sacred
pages of my
self-care journal;
i ink the poetry
of my own
well-being—a
testament to the
art of nurturing
the nurturer

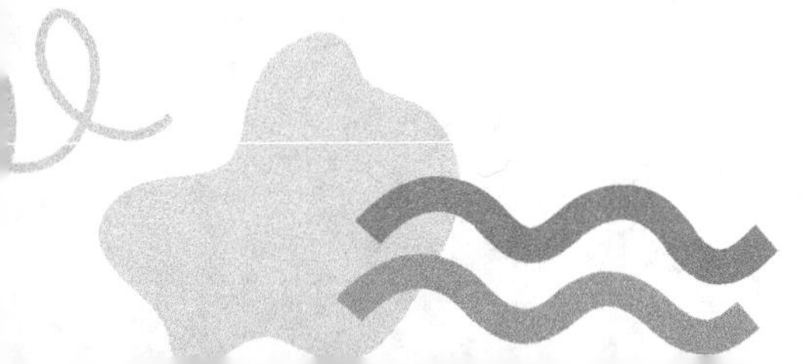

As a mother, keeping a self-care notebook has been my haven in the lovely chaos of everyday existence. It's a mirror that reflects back the subtleties of my wellbeing, more than just a book of pages.

Every submission turns into a celebration of the little things in life—those intentionally self-loving gestures, those snatched moments of loneliness, and the laughter shared with loved ones.

The pages serve as a canvas for the colours of my emotions, a compass that points me back toward my own needs, and a repository for the echo of my reflections.

This journal is about reclamation, not simply recording. It gives me the confidence to set aside time for self-care, write down my goals, and watch as fleeting moments turn into treasured memories.

CALL YOUR

Best Friend

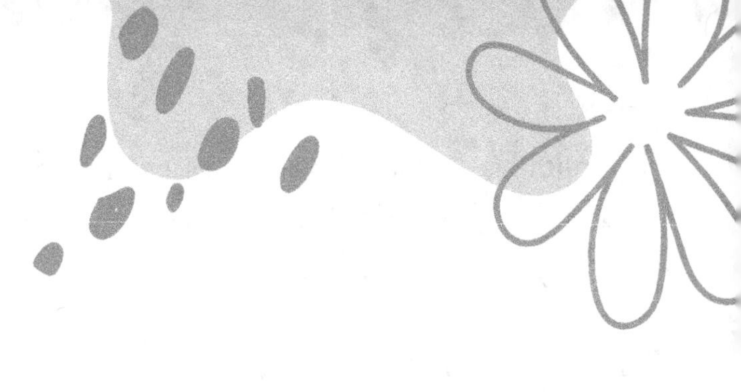

in the dance of motherhood; a call to your best friend is the music that soothes the soul

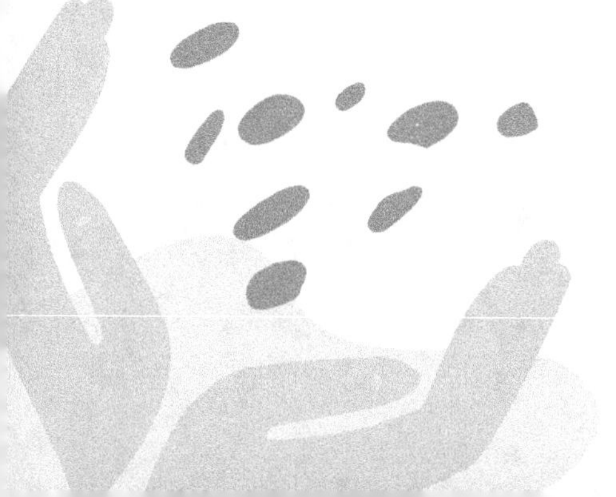

Sometimes, in the chaos of parenthood, all it takes is a quick phone call to your closest friend to help you stay grounded.

It's more than simply a discussion; it's a place where understanding and humour are allowed to flow freely and a lifeline to sanity.

The voice on the other end of the line becomes a source of strength and renewal in those fleeting minutes between naps and supper preparation.

This call serves as a reminder that, during diaper mayhem and bedtime stories, your best friend is a lifeline, a confidante, and a fellow warrior.

You share the highs, lows, and everything in between.

DISTRACTION FREE

Coffee

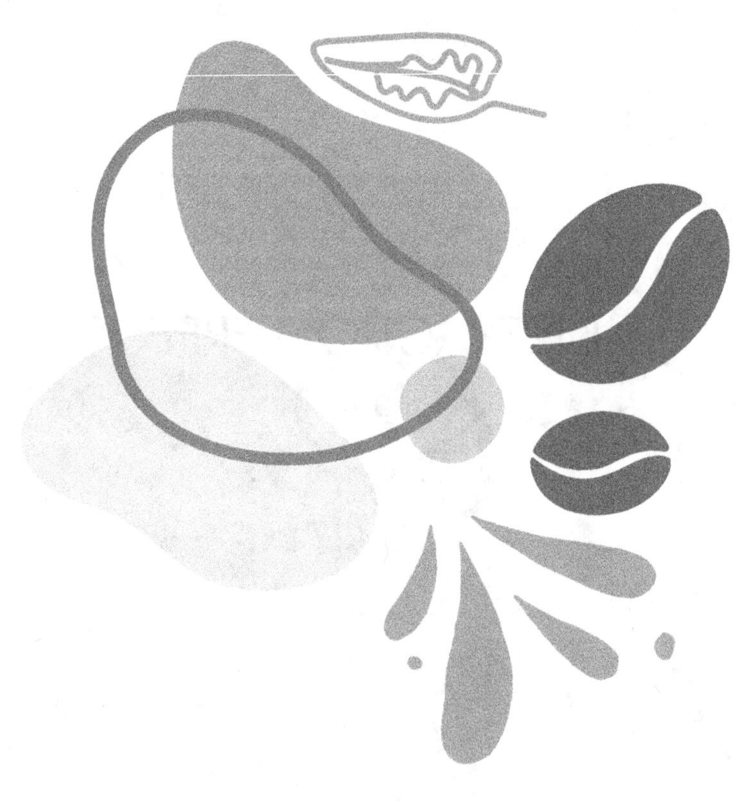

in the hush of dawn; a cup of coffee becomes more than a beverage; it's a quiet rebellion against the chaos of the day

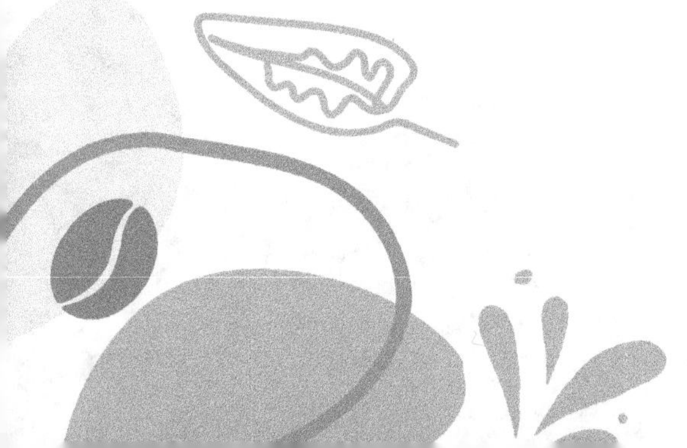

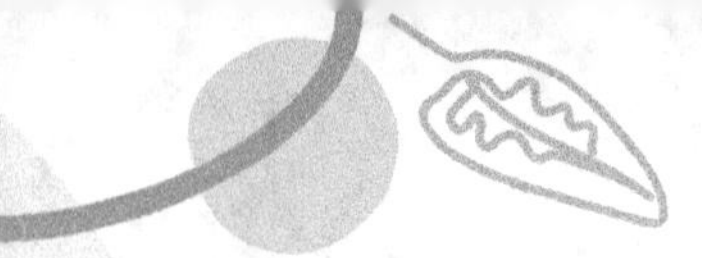

Only fifteen minutes earlier, when the world is still asleep and the day has not yet begun to unveil its demands, is a magical moment.

The smell of freshly made coffee becomes a companion to your thoughts in this peaceful window, providing a peaceful time.

The day's distractions go as you hold that warm mug in your arms, letting you enjoy every sip in peaceful tranquillity.

It's more than simply coffee; it's a self-care ritual and a tiny protest against the busyness of life. So, get up a little earlier, make the sunrise your friend, and savour those quiet minutes with your favourite beverage.

Conclusion

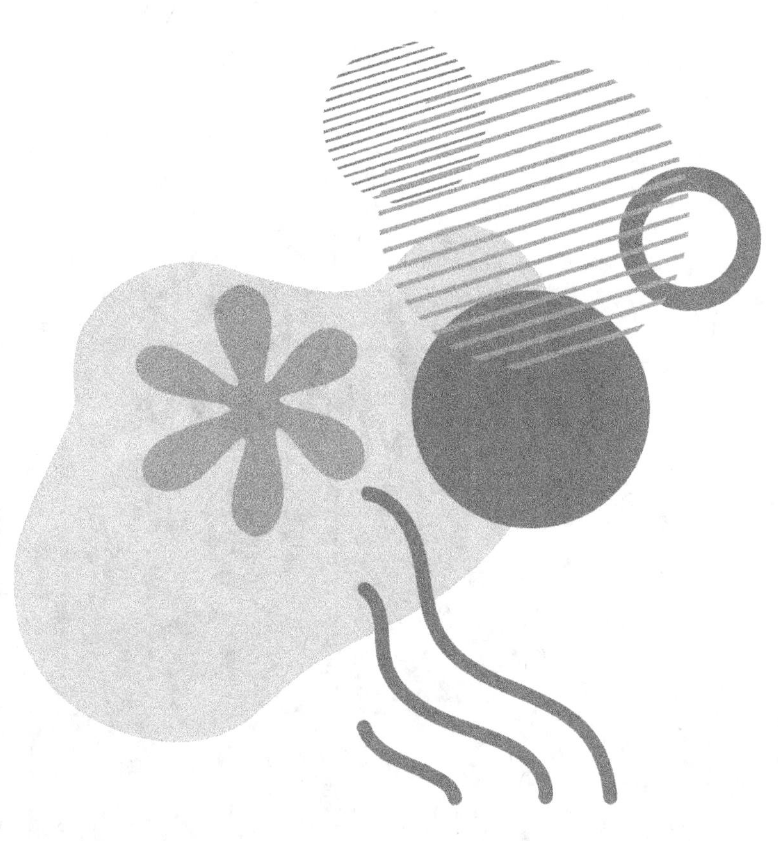

I hope you have enjoyed this book mama, sometimes all we need is one idea to get us going. Remember you are doing so well, we have to be grateful for the small wins as well; just by getting out of bed, having a shower, making a home cooked meal, or raising your happy healthy baby! Don't have high expectations. Believe in yourself and it's ok to say no, we don't realise how much that word can mean to keeping ourselves well looked after.

WHAT DID YOU LEARN?

I discovered that gentle accumulation of heartfelt moments—rather than huge gestures—is what matters most when it comes to self-care for mothers. Crafting, taking thoughtful breaks, exploring new cuisine, and taking up new hobbies are more than just pastimes; they're hints of self-love. What did I learn? For me, self-care consists of a patchwork of tiny, deliberate actions; it's a continuous conversation with my own health and a creative dance with the demands of parenting. It serves as a reminder that by taking care of myself, I can better take care of other people.

MOVING FORWARD

As we conclude this exploration of self-care for mums, it's not the end but a stepping stone into an ongoing journey. Moving forward, let's carry the essence of these self-care practices with us, weaving them into the fabric of our daily lives. May crafting, mindful moments, culinary adventures, and new hobbies be not just occasional retreats but cherished rituals.

This is an invitation to embrace self-care as a constant companion, an ally in the ebb and flow of motherhood. Let's move forward with the understanding that nurturing ourselves isn't a luxury; it's a necessity. As we navigate the beautiful chaos ahead, may self-care be the compass guiding us to moments of joy, resilience, and a deeper connection with our own well-being. The journey continues, and so does the celebration of the incredible mothers we are.

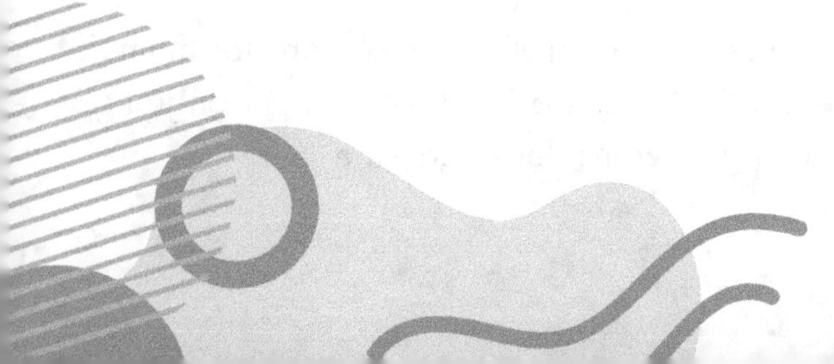